Healthy Homemade Baby Purees

Easy, Organic, Nutritious Food Recipes For
Healthy Babies

PENNY REYNOLDS

ISBN-13:978-1518864735

ISBN-10:1518864732

DEDICATION

To my mum, Carlota; you're the best!

TABLE OF CONTENTS

INTRODUCTION

Preparing homemade baby food is easier than you think. It is akin to cooking your regular simple, nutritious and healthy meals; only this time, it is modified to the appropriate texture for your baby, with hygiene and safety concerns being uppermost in your mind.

At about 6 months, your baby is ready to try homemade foods. From holding her head up by herself, to no longer automatically sticking out her tongue, eyeing meals and reaching for your plate, your baby is telling you that she wants more than just milk.

Start with rice cereals then proceed to one-fruit or vegetable purees such as pear, apple, peas and potato. This will help you to detect the cause of your baby's allergic, if she has one. It is also advisable to introduce a new food to your baby in the morning so you could watch for any allergic reaction in the course of the day. Do not introduce new foods everyday but give one or two day's interval before trying something else. After a while, you will be able to try a mix of fruits, vegetables, and more solid meals.

Preparing and cooking your baby's food is a simple process that need not take up a lot of time and expense. You will even begin to enjoy it and look forward to it as you make a wide range of baby food flavors by mixing and matching various fruit and vegetable cubes.

Homemade Purees Vs Store-bought Foods

Homemade baby foods are healthier than jar foods obtained from grocery stores. Fresh fruits and vegetables are used in preparing purees for your baby. Even more solid homemade baby foods are devoid of addictives, thickeners, salt and sugar that characterize commercial foods. You are then left with natural, organic, nutritious and healthy foods for your baby.

Manufacturers want their commercial foods to last long so they pass them through intense heat for shelf life extension and for sterilization. This process leads to loss of some nutrients, aromas, and flavors, leaving you with bland-tasting and unnatural purees. This also goes to show that your store bought jars are much older than your baby! Purees prepared at home are fresh and have a more authentic taste since the natural flavor and taste of the vegetables are still intact.

With homemade baby foods, you are in control; you can provide your baby with the specific nutrients that are needed. For instance, if your baby comes down with a cold, you can make a puree packed with vitamin C. For constipation; pear, papaya, peaches and peas are of great help. Beans, spinach or beef also provides your baby with the iron that she needs.

Having been accustomed to taking homemade food, your baby will find it easier to make the shift to eating and enjoying family food prepared at home. However, if the baby relies solely on jar foods, it will be difficult to feed her with natural and wholesome foods when the time comes, without a big fuss. So what you are really doing is training her taste buds and helping her get used to the variety of flavors that await her.

Versatility of the meals is also another strong point. There is a wide variety of fruit and vegetables to choose and combine, presenting your baby with a whole new different taste at all times. As the baby grows older, you could also vary the texture of the purees from very smooth to coarse, tantalizing her taste buds and providing her with a new eating experience from time to time. Commercial foods lack the flavor and texture that is available in homemade foods. They are bland. And let's not also forget the economic benefit. You save up of lots of money by preparing foods in batches.

While pre-packaged baby foods are convenient and handy, they should be used as minimally as possible, such as during emergencies, when you are away from home or as part of a larger meal.

How To Start

Start with a spoonful or two of:

- Pureed or mashed fruits, like cooked apple, banana, or pear.
- Pureed or mashed cooked veggies like as carrot, potato or parsnip.
- Gluten-free cereal like baby rice, maize, millet and cornmeal, mixed with your baby's regular milk.

Once your baby happily accepts these foods, be prepared to move her to other foods like meat, fish, pastas, rice, potatoes and beans. But do not expect her to gobble up all her food once she begins to eat as she can only take tiny portions for her tiny tummy! Breast milk or formula will still play a major part of her nutrition for months to come. Feed her with at least 2 to 2½ cups of formula or milk every day

As you offer your baby her first spoon, remember that it is a brand new experience for her so you will need to be patient, especially as it can get pretty messy. Both of you should sit comfortably and then you give her small servings. Increase it only when she indicates interest. Do not force her to eat but try again the next day.

Food Safety Tips

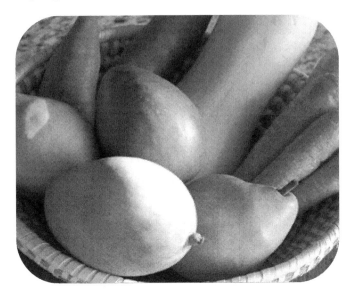

The first safety tip is to ensure that your hands, all utensils, work space and ingredients are extremely clean before cooking. Wash fruits and vegetables with cold, running water. Keep all kitchen tools, equipment and counters clean. Sponges, cloths and towels must also be spotless. Wooden cutting boards are likely to harbor bacteria so use glass or plastic ones. This is worth re-emphasizing as many parents take it for granted: always wash your hands before you begin any kitchen task.

Refrigerate chicken, fish and raw meat separately to avoid contamination with other foods. After cooking, wash cutting boards, plates, utensils, counters, and any other thing that have come in contact with the raw juices. Cook chicken, meat, fish and eggs thoroughly. To prevent germs from breeding in between temperatures, hot foods must always be kept hot and colds foods cold. Cool prepared homemade foods immediately to prevent the growth of bacteria.

Do not feed your baby any food that has been left to sit at room temperature for more than 2 hours. Throw out such foods immediately. Additionally, discard foods your baby does not finish. Once her spoon has touched her mouth and gone back to the food, bacteria will multiply. Discard leftovers that have been heated up once and jar or containers you have fed your baby from. Make sure the cans and jars you use to store foods have working seals.

Freezing& Defrosting Baby Foods

Homemade baby foods are usually prepared in bulk so there is need to safely store them in ice-cube trays and other containers and then place in the refrigerators or freezers for consumption at a later time.

Sterilize your regular ice-cube trays/containers before using them by pouring boiling water over them. Clean thoroughly and then ladle your homemade baby food into each section. The tray should have a lid to prevent infiltration from the odors of other foods in the freezer and to protect the food from freezer burn. A food-safe plastic wrap can also be used to cover the tray if it has no lid. Do not use foil because some pieces of it could enter into the food unknowingly.

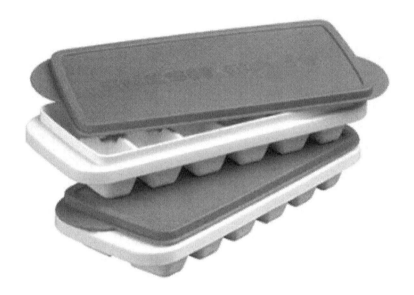

Put the ice-cube tray in the freezer and when the cubes are frozen, press them out with a blunt knife and remove to freezer containers or zip-top bags, which take up less space in your freezer. Label and date them. Now you have about an ounce sized of little portions of baby food. At first one cube will be sufficient for one meal but as your baby grows older, you could store larger quantities in larger plastic containers or simply place 2 cubes in each zip-top bag.

Other ways of freezing baby food is to use silicone mini-muffin pans or spoon it into freezer-safe jars and place the jars directly in the freezer. Avoid using glass, except of course, the manufacturer specifically states on the packaging that it is safe to do so. You wouldn't want the jar to break or crack and drop tiny glass shards into your baby's food!

To defrost the frozen food a day before use, transfer it food from the freezer to the refrigerator or use the defrost setting on your microwave. But, if you are going to use the food within 24 hours of preparing it, cool quickly, within 90 minutes, and then store in the fridge. To speed up cooling, sit the bowl in a pan of cold water or spread food out in a shallow bowl or container. Anything that you wouldn't be using within 24 hours should be frozen. Individually portioned baby food can be stored in the freezer for up to a month.

Do not refreeze baby food that has been defrosted. Reheat baby food until it is piping hot all through with steam coming out. Let it cool down before you offer the baby though. Place a tiny bit of food on the back of your hand or the inside of your wrist to assess the temperature before offering the baby. For purees that don't need reheating, such as fruit purees; check that these are fully defrosted before giving them to your baby. If you are using a microwave to heat food up, stir thoroughly to avoid hot spots.

Preparing Baby Food

When preparing your baby's first foods, be sure to start with foods that will not put your baby at risk of harm by choking or resulting in allergies. Before you begin to cook, make sure all bones, seeds, core and fats have been removed. Since the skins of most fruits and veggies have much of their nutritional value, you could choose to cook and puree the vegetables with their skins on or remove them just before pureeing. For convenience, prepare different types of foods and store them for later use.

There are 3 best methods for cooking baby food. These include:

Steaming:

Steaming in small amounts of water will retain most of the nutrients in the food. Of all cooking methods, this is the best. Do not overcook the food though; otherwise it will become waterlogged and unpleasing to the taste. What is ideal is to add a little of the steamed water to it; this way, you will be incorporating some of the lost nutrients back into the baby's food. Even if you choose to go the way of boiling, you should still boil with little water and keep any remaining water from the cooked food.

Microwaving

Cooking baby food in a microwave makes it easier to cook small amounts well. Microwaving large amounts can lead to uneven cooking. Check your food to ensure it is evenly cooked before pureeing otherwise your baby may be unable to swallow the resulting roughly texture of an uneven cooked food.

Dry Baking

Dry baking is baking without oil. It helps to intensify the flavors of vegetables with just a liquid added in the course of puréeing the vegetables. Carrots, potato, sweet potato, parsnips and corn are some of these veggies. However, if you bake meat, puree it with a little water and not the meat juices because juices may heighten the taste and this will be too strong for the baby.

Cooking methods you should avoid: frying and grilling.

These cooking methods do not retain nutrients. It is also not safe for the baby to consume oil from frying and the amounts of carbon from grilling.

What To Avoid

Babies love the natural flavors of foods. Avoid addictives like salt, sugar, oil and honey. Why?

- A baby's kidney is not developed enough for salt and sodium. Do not add salt to her foods.
- Naturally sweet fruits do not need to be sweetened with sugar. You wouldn't want your baby to experience baby tooth decay!
- Add honey to foods only when the baby is at least 12 months old to avoid infant botulism. At this age, the baby's digestive system is strong enough to cope with the bacteria.

Some cheese varieties and unpasteurized cheeses like goat's cheese, blue cheese and brie should be avoided.

Also, do not give your baby, shellfish or raw or semi cooked egg to avoid food poisoning.

Avoid all fatty foods, spicy foods, foods with artificial colorings and flavors, foods with preservatives like sulfates and nitrates and all fried foods. Let your baby enjoy food as naturally as possible.

Organic Fruit Purees For Beginners (6-7 Months)

Fruit purees are the perfect first foods for your baby. All it takes is to cook a little organic fruit until it is soft, then puree until thoroughly smooth.

Your baby can take it immediately or you can store it by freezing them in ice cube trays. These fruit cubes can then be taken as desserts or even mixed with the baby's cereal.

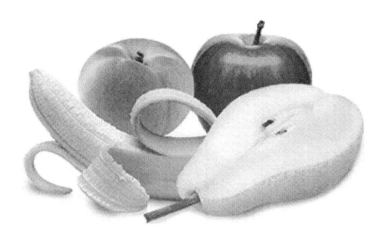

Pureed Banana

This recipe contains vitamins A and C, minerals and folate.

<u>Ingredients</u>

1 ripe banana

<u>Preparation</u>

1. Peel and puree the banana or mash with a fork.

2. Cook 25 seconds in the microwave to soften.

3. Add water, breast milk or formula if too thick. Add cereal if too thin.

Pureed Avocado

Just like banana, there is no need to cook this healthy fruit recipe.

1 ripe avocado

Preparation

1. Peel avocado and take out the pit.

2. Cut it out, mash with fork and feed baby.

One Day Apple
Ingredients:

3 medium-sized apples, chopped

½ cup of water

1/8 teaspoon of cinnamon (optional)

Preparation

1. Peel apples and cut into cubes of about 1 inch. Discard the core.

2. Place the apples in a saucepan with water, add cinnamon if using and simmer10-12 minutes on medium-low heat until tender.

3. Add all contents of pan to food processor and puree until smooth. If necessary, add water.

4. Distribute evenly into ice cube trays and freeze until solid.

Peary Plum

Serves: 6 portions

Ingredients

1 pear, peeled, cored & cut into quarters

2 plums, peeled, stone removed &cut into halves

Preparation

1. Place fruit in a steamer and cook until tender, about 5 minutes.

2. Purée and add baby's regular milk or boiled water. Mix well until smooth.

Perfect Pears

Simple, delicious and nutritious: just the perfect first food for your baby.

Ingredients:

2 or 3 ripe medium-sized pears, chopped

½ cup of water

Preparation:

1. Chop the pears into squares of about ¼ inch. Discard the peel and core.

2. Next, place the pears in a saucepan, add the water and simmer for 10-12 minutes on medium-low heat until the pears are tender.

3. Add the contents to a food processor and puree until smooth. If necessary, add water. Distribute evenly into ice cube trays and place in the freezer until solid.

Organic Fruit Purees For Beginners (6-8Months)

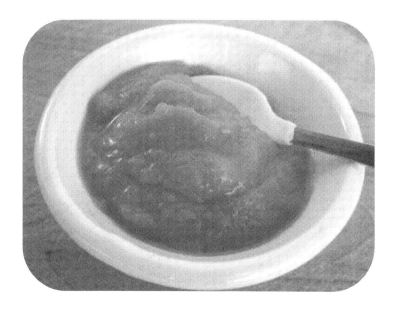

Mango Relish

Rich in vitamins A,E, K and C, folate, minerals, calcium, sodium, potassium and magnesium.

<u>Ingredients</u>

1 ripe mango

Water, formula or breast milk

<u>Preparation</u>

1. Peel mango and cut in half, deseed, and mango into chunks.

2. Puree in a blender or food processor and add the desired liquid to attain the right consistency.

Apricot Puree

This contains vitamins A, C, folate, calcium, potassium and phosphorus.

Ingredients

1 pound of dried apricots

2 cups of apple juice, white grape juice or pear juice

Preparation

1. Bring fruit and liquid to a boil; simmer 15 minutes while reserving liquid for the puree.

2. Puree mixture and add the liquid to get a smooth puree.

3. To thicken up, add cereal (if desired). Pour into cubes and freeze.

Papaya Puree

Papaya can be taken raw if ripe.

Ingredients

1 ripe papaya

Water, formula or breast milk

Preparation

1. Peel papaya, deseed and cut into chunks.

2. Puree and add water, breast milk or formula. If too thin, add cereal.

3. If your baby doesn't take to raw food, steam the cut papaya gently for 5 to 10 minutes before pureeing.

Apple, Pear, Banana Mush

Serves: 6 portions

1 pear, peeled, cored& diced

1 ripe banana

1 apple, peeled, cored& diced

2 tablespoons of baby's regular milk

Preparation

1. Put the diced apple and pear into a saucepan and add water to cover it.

2. Cook over a low heat until softened, about 8 – 10 minute.

3. Pour into a food processor. Add the banana and milk and then purée until smooth.

Baked Apples

Ingredients

Apple

Butter

Cinnamon

Preparation

1. Core the apple but leave the peel on.

2. On the inside of the apple, place a little amount of butter and sprinkle cinnamon over.

3. Place the apple in a pan with about 1 inch of water to cover apples slightly.

15

4. Bake until tender or for about 30 minutes at 400-degree F, checking the water level.

5. Mash the baked apple or cut the baked apple into bits and serve as a finger food.

Banana Applesauce
<u>Ingredients</u>

1 ripe banana

1 apple

<u>Preparation</u>

1. Peel apple, core and cut into chunks/ slices.

2. Place into a pan and add water to cover apples slightly. Boil until tender.

3. Puree apple to achieve a smooth applesauce consistency.

4. Peel banana and mash with a fork. Heat the banana in the microwave for 20 seconds to soften it up, if needed.

5. Add applesauce to the banana. (If your baby is at least 8 months, sprinkle with crushed cheerios or wheat germ).

6. Puree or mash with a potato masher for smoothness.

Papaya Mango Pear Puree

Papaya, mango and pear combo not only sound delicious but taste so as well. It's worth giving it a go. Besides, it helps to relive constipation by softening baby's stools and relieving discomfort.

Serves: 12-24 portions

Ingredients

1 mango, diced

½ papaya, seeded, skin removed, diced

3 apricots, cored &diced

3 pears, peeled, cored& diced

1 cup water

Preparation

1. In a medium saucepan, heat the water and add the fruits.

2. Simmer 8-10 minutes or until soft.

3. Blend together the softened fruits, adding the cooking water until desired consistency is attained.

Apple, Pear & Cinnamon Purée
Serves: 6 portions

Ingredients

2 ripe pears

2 apples

4 tablespoons of pure unsweetened apple juice or water

A pinch of ground cinnamon (optional)

<u>Preparation</u>

1. Peel the fruit and place in a saucepan.

2. Add the apple juice or water and cinnamon, if using.

3. Cover and cook over low heats until fruit is tender, about 6 to 8 minute.

4. Blend the fruit to desired consistency.

Baked Baby Peaches

1 peach

Water

<u>Preparation</u>

1. Cut the peach in half and deseed.

2. Add 1 inch water to a pan and then place the cut peach side down in it.

3. Bake at 400 degrees Fahrenheit until the skin crumples.

4. Remove the skin and reserve the extra water for thinning the puree.

Apple, Pear And Peach Delight

<u>Ingredients</u>

2 ripe peaches

1 ripe pear, diced

1 sweet apple, diced

2 tablespoon water

<u>Preparation</u>

1. Cut a cross at the top and bottom of the peaches and place in a heat-proof bowl.

2. Pour boiling water over it, let it sit for 30 seconds and then pour cold water to peel off the skin.

3. Cut peaches in fourth, remove pit and dice. Add to saucepan together with the pear, apples and water.

4. Boil, simmer on low heat and cook until fruit is soft, about 10 minutes.

5. Cool, puree until smooth, adding water if too thick. Freeze in portions and thaw 1-2 hours before serving.

Vegetable Purees (6-8months+)

Some babies may prefer fruit purees to vegetables on account of its sweet taste. However, vegetables like pumpkin and peas are sweet-tasting and contain essential vitamins like all veggies. To retain most of their nutrients, vegetables are better steamed. This also helps to soften them and achieve a pulpy texture for the baby.

You could try to experiment by combining 2-3 vegetables or fruits and altering the texture as you go along.

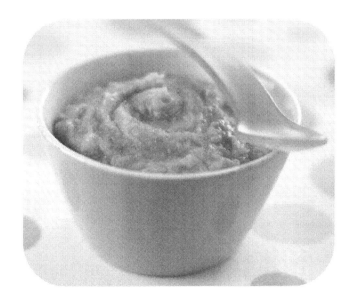

Garden Veggie Combo

This combo is a delightful mix of carrots, green beans, peas and summer squash

1. Cover all the vegetables with water and boil until tender.

2. Reserve the water for later use

3. Puree everything in a blender or food processor, adding the reserved water when necessary.

Carrot & Parsnip

Serves: 5 portions

Ingredients

1 parsnip, peeled& chopped

2 carrots, peeled& chopped

Preparation

1. Steam the veggies until tender or for about 20 minutes.

2. Blend to a purée, adding some of your baby's regular milk or some of the boiled water at the bottom of the steamer to make the purée thinner.

Squash Medley

Butternut squash, Hubbard squash, winter squash and acorn squash can be combined to make this healthy recipe for your child.

Preparation

1. Cut squash in half, deseed and place side down on a baking sheet with an inch water.

2. Cook 40 minutes at 400 degrees F but keep checking the water level.

3. Once the shell puckers, scrape out the meat from it and puree; add water to attain the right consistency.

4. Alternatively, chunk and boil squash and then remove the meat when the skin becomes tender.

Green Beans Day

<u>Ingredients</u>

1 lb. fresh green beans, washed, ends snap & cut into pieces

½ cup of water

<u>Preparation</u>

1. Steam the beans in the water until tender, about 7-8 minutes (Check the water level constantly)

2. Reserve the leftover water for thinning the beans if necessary.

Pea Puree

Peas are highly nutritious. They are rich in vitamin A, C, and iron. They can even help prevent cancer.

1pound of pea pods = about 1 cup of peas.

1. Cut off the top and bottom of the pod and then open the pod by pulling the string

2. Remove the peas by pushing your thumb along the inside of the pod.

3. Rinse the peas in a colander and then steam or boil to help knock the little stems off.

<u>Preparation</u>

1. Steam 3-5 minutes until tender.

2. Blend with a little water from the pot.

3. Serve cooked peas as finger foods for babies over 9 months old

Apple & Sweet Potato

Serves: 4 portions

Ingredients

2 sweet potatoes, peeled

2 apples, peeled& cored

Preparation

1. Steam together the sweet potatoes and apples until tender.

2. Purée until smooth, adding milk or water, if necessary to thin the puree.

Pumpkin Puree

This is rich in vitamins, folate, niacin, calcium, minerals iron, potassium and magnesium.

Ingredients

1 small sugar pumpkin (less than 5 lb)

Preparation

1. Cut pumpkin into two, deseed and place face down on a baking sheet with 1 inch water.

2. Bake for 40 minutes at 400 degrees F, keeping water level up.

3. Remove the 'meat' of the pumpkin and puree, adding water to attain the right consistency.

4. Alternatively, boil the cut pumpkin in water and take out the skin when the meat is soft and tender.

3. Puree cooked beans in a food processor and thin with the steam water to get the right consistency for your baby.

3. Let it cool and then evenly distribute amongst cupcake tins or ice cube trays.

Cheesy Leek, Cauliflower& Sweet Potato
Ingredients

1tseaspoon of butter

1/8 cup of peas

1 small carrot diced

½ small onion, chopped

1 small potato diced

2 medium broccoli florets cut small

1/8 cup of cheese, grated

Baby's usual milk (optional)

Preparation

1. Fry the onion in the butter in a saucepan for 3-4 minutes and set aside. Add together the carrot and potato in another pan and simmer in little water until vegetables are cooked, about 15 minutes.

2. Add the cut broccoli and cook 5 more minutes. Add the peas and cook for several seconds.

3. Remove, add the onion and milk and mash smoothly. Stir in the cheese, cool and serve.

Carrot, Broccoli & Potato

Serves: 4 portions

Ingredients

1 carrot

½ cup broccoli floret

1 large potato

Preparation

1. Peel and chop the carrot, broccoli and potato.

2. Add all chopped vegetables to a pan, cover with water and bring to a boil. Simmer about 20 minutes.

3. Blend the vegetables to make a smooth baby purée.

Butternut Squash & Pear

Serves: 5 portions

Ingredients

1 ripe pear, peeled, cored& chopped

1 medium butternut squash, peeled& sliced in half

Preparation

1. Remove the seeds of the peeled and sliced butternut squash, chop into pieces and steam for 12 minutes.

2. Add to the pear to the steamer and keep cooking until the squash is tender or for about for 5 minutes. Puree in a blender.

Sweet Potato And Plantains Puree

<u>Ingredients</u>

1 cup sweet potato, cooked & mashed

1 plantain, peeled & chopped

¼ cup formula or breast milk

¾ cup low sodium chicken stock

1 tsp fresh, chopped parsley

¼ cup plain organic yoghurt

Pinch of pepper

<u>Preparation</u>

1. Boil the plantain in the chicken broth; simmer 10 minutes until the plantain is soft.

2. Drain mixture but reserve the cooking liquid.

3. Combine all ingredients in a blender or food processor, adding a little water if too thick.

4. Puree and warm to proper temperature.

Sweet Potato And Spinach Puree

Do not feed your baby spinach alone as it may pose some problems. For your baby to enjoy its rich iron content, spinach must be combined with other vegetables like carrots, pumpkin or sweet potato. You may also add a sweet fruit to vary the taste of the meal.

<u>Ingredients</u>

1 sweet potato

Handful sprigs or leaves of spinach, cut& washed

Preparation

1. Boil the sweet potato in water until done. Peel the cooked potato and mash with a fork until smooth.

2. Steam the cut and washed spinach leaves until soft. Add it to the mashed potato, mixing well.

3. Serve when done. The sweetness of the potato will override the blandness of the spinach. Your baby wouldn't notice.

4. Alternatively, make a fruit-veggie medley by adding an apple. Steam or bake the diced sweet potato, mash with the cooked apple. You may be amazed at how much your baby will love it!

Carrot & Pea

Make a smooth puree by adding baby milk to this recipe.

Serves: 4 portions

Ingredients

½ oz frozen peas

2 carrots

Preparation

1. Peel carrots and cut them into pieces. Place in a pan and cover it with boiling water. Cook 15 -20 minutes.

2. Add the peas and cook another 5 minutes.

3. Blend the vegetables in a food processor and add to your baby's usual milk.

Butternut Squash & Carrot

<u>Ingredients</u>

1/2 butternut squash, peeled & chopped

1 carrot, peeled & chopped

2 tablespoons milk

2 tablespoons baby rice

<u>Preparation</u>

1. Steam carrot and butternut squash until tender or for 15 to 20 minutes.

2. Puree, add milk and baby rice. Serves: 4 portions

Veggie Medley

<u>Ingredients</u>

A few florets of broccoli

1 small carrot

1 sweet potato

1 handful of green beans

<u>Preparation</u>

1. Steam vegetables till soft and tender. Boil root vegetable separately. Blend with a hand blender with some cool boiled water.

2. Scoop out and serve your baby when cool.

3. To thicken the consistency, add cooked mashed rice or oatmeal

4. You may also thin it by adding vegetable or chicken stock and convert the mix to soup.

Butternut Squash & Pear

Serves: 5 portions

Ingredients

1 ripe pear

1 medium butternut squash

Preparation

1. Peel and slice the butternut squash in half. Deseed; chop into cubes and steam 12-15 minutes.

2. Peel the pear, core and chop it and add to the steamer. Cook until the squash is tender, about 5 to 8 minutes.

3. Once tender, puree mixture in a blender until smooth.

Zucchini Or Summer Squash

Squash or zucchini, narrow in diameter

Preparation

1. Wash and peel with potato peeler. Cut squash into chunks.

2. Steam until the chunks are tender and then puree.

3. Add water to get the right consistency.

Yams Or Sweet Potato

Rich in vitamins A, C, folate, sodium, magnesium, phosphorus and calcium, your baby will love this.

Yams or sweet potatoes, washed and poked with holes

Preparation

1. Wrap in tin foil and place in the microwave, cooking for 8 minutes until tender.

2. place in the oven and cook at 400 degrees F for about 30 minutes.

3. Remove skin from potatoes or yam, puree the flesh and add water to desired consistency.

Potatoes And Pumpkin With Apple Snack
Ingredients

1 small potato

1-2 apples

¼ of a small pumpkin

Pinch of nutmeg

Preparation

1. Peel and dice all the vegetables and simmer in water until tender.

2. Drain the vegetables while reserving the water.

3. Add everything, including the nutmeg to a food processor and puree.

4. Add the reserve water until the desired thickness is attained.

Cereals (6-7 Months+)

Oats, brown rice, baby rice, buckwheat, barley, cornmeal and other gluten-free cereals are the perfect weaning foods for your baby. They are non allergic-causing food as well, so you do not need to be concerned about allergies. Nevertheless, introduce wheat to your baby only when he or she has accepted all other cereals.

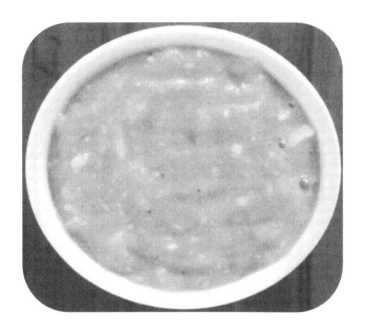

Brown Rice With Apple & Cinnamon
Ingredients

1 tablespoon of brown rice

4-5 oz formula or breast milk

1 small apple pureed

Pinch of cinnamon, ground

Filtered water, if necessary

<u>Preparation</u>

1. Ground the brown rice until it is in powdery form. Add some milk and mix well. Add the remaining milk and cook until creamy, about 10 minutes.

2. Add the pureed apple and cinnamon powder. Let it cool and then serve.

Brown Rice Cereal

Brown rice is better than white rice. It is rich in vitamins B, iron, fiber, manganese and flavor.

<u>Ingredients</u>

1/4 cup of rice powder (brown rice ground in food processor or blender)

1 cup of water

<u>Preparation</u>

1. Add water to saucepan and bring to boil. Add the rice powder and stir often.

2. Simmer for 10 minutes while whisking often.

3. Add breast milk, formula or fruits if desired. Serve warm.

Oatmeal Cereal
<u>Ingredients</u>

1/4 cups of ground oats (do not use Quick Cook or instant)

3/4 cup of water

<u>Preparation</u>

1. Add water to saucepan and bring to boil. Add the ground oats and stir often.

2. Simmer for 10 minutes while whisking often.

3. Add breast milk, formula or fruits if desired. Serve warm.

Barley With Kiwi & Banana

Barley is rich in protein and folate. When grounded, it is ideal for cereals but older kids can enjoy cooked grains without milling in soups.

Ingredients

1 ripe kiwi fruit

1 ripe banana

2 tablespoons of barley grains or milled

Milk or water (optional)

Preparation

1. Put the ground barley in a pan of water and cook15 minutes, whisking constantly to prevent it from sticking to pot.

2. Mash the banana and kiwi in a bowl. Add the pureed fruit to the barley and then stir well.

3. Add a little milk, if using.

Millet And Apple Cereal

Millet is a versatile grain and can be used as a replacement for rice dishes. It is rich in minerals and vitamins. It also makes good breakfast porridge with fruits when used in its powdered form.

Ingredients

1 ripe apple

Vegetable oil

½ tablespoon millet grain

Pinch cinnamon powder

Water

Preparation

1. Add a little oil to a pan and then toast the millet grains until brownish.

2. Add water, bring to a boil and simmer over low heat until the grains are soft and fluff, and water has been absorbed.

3. Serve on its own sprinkled with cinnamon or add any fruit puree such as apple, melon and pear to vary the taste. Vegetable purees like mashed pumpkin or pureed carrots can also be substituted for the fruit purees.

Banana Oatmeal With Blueberries

This recipe contains vitamins A and C, fiber and antioxidants that your baby needs.

Ingredients

1tablespooon organic blueberries

½ of a ripe small banana

¼ cup of plain oatmeal

1 tablespoon whole milk yoghurt

Preparation

1. Add oats to pan then add water and cook.

2. Once cooked, add yogurt to the cooked oats and transfer to a blender.

3. Add blueberries and bananas to the mixture and blend until thoroughly smooth.

Ground Barley Cereal
Ingredients

1/4 cup of ground barley

1 cup water

Preparation

1. Add water to saucepan and bring to boil. Add the barley.

2. Simmer for 10 minutes while whisking often.

3. Add breast milk, formula or fruits if desired. Serve warm.

Fine Buckwheat Oatmeal

Buckwheat is high in minerals and vitamins. Contrary to its name, it is neither from the wheat family nor considered a grain. It is generally milled for faster and easier cooking.

Ingredients

2 tablespoons of fine buckwheat flour

11/4 cups of breast milk or formula milk

Preparation

1. In a saucepan, warm the milk and then add the flour. Cook on medium heat for 8- 10 minutes until smooth.

2. Cool and then serve. If too thick, add more milk.

3. To vary the taste and texture, add a fruit like banana.

Banana And Oats Cereal

Oats contain B vitamins, fiber and calcium. Rolled oats are more beneficial than quick or instant oats. However, it may contain traces of gluten; consequently, you should consult your pediatrician if your family has a history of allergy.

Ingredients

1 small banana, mashed

½ tablespoon oats

Water

Preparation

1. Ground the oats in blender. Cook the ground oats in a pan of water, stirring often to prevent clumping until soft. Keep stirring while simmering to prevent sticking.

2. Cook until it is like the consistency of porridge. Add the banana to the porridge and serve your baby.

3. For more variety, try using millet instead of oatmeal.

Chicken & Turkey Recipes (9-12 Months+)

Cook meats until they lose their pink color in the middle.

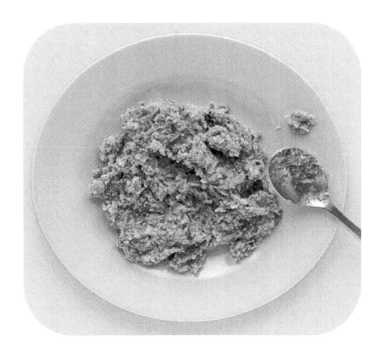

Flavorful Chicken Casserole

This carefully flavored recipe is an excellent source of iron, with vitamin C and beta-carotene.

Ingredients

1 chicken breast, skinned & diced

½ an onion, finely chopped

1 carrot, peeled & diced

1 dessertspoon olive oil

3 or 4 button mushrooms, wiped& thinly sliced

1 bouquet garni

1/3 cup of frozen peas, thawed

5 ounce of water

<u>Preparation</u>

1. Fry the onion and chicken gently in the oil until the chicken is thoroughly cooked on all sides.

2. Add the mushrooms, carrot and bouquet garni. Stir well and add the water. Cover and gently simmer for 15 minutes and then add the peas.

3. Cook for 5 minutes to warm the peas through. Remove the bouquet garni .

4. Blend to the right consistency for your baby.

Chicken With Apple& Carrots Purée

Your baby will take to this tasty chicken purée recipe. The apple and carrots add flavor and sweetness to the chicken, giving it a smooth swallow-able texture.

Servings: 5 portions

<u>Ingredients</u>

12oz carrots, peeled & sliced

1/2 small onion, peeled &chopped

1, 4oz chicken breast, cut into pieces

1/2 tbsp olive oil

1 small apple, cored, peeled & chopped

8 fl oz unsalted chicken stock or water with 1 bay leaf

<u>Preparation</u>

1. Sauté onion in heated olive oil until softened.

2. Add the carrots, chicken stock or water with bay leaf and bring to a boil.

3. Lower heat, cover and cook 10 minutes. Add the chicken pieces and apple to the carrots, and cook another10 minutes.

4. Remove bay leaf, if using. Puree all and serve lukewarm. Freeze leftover in individual portions.

Apricot Sweet Chicken

Fruit, chicken and sweet potato is all combined in this meal to provide your baby with the required nutrients.

<u>Ingredients</u>

1 small chicken thigh, diced into small pieces

2 fresh apricots, wash, cut into halves, stones removed and then cut into quarters

1 cup sweet potato, chopped

1 tablespoons olive oil

1 cup water

<u>Preparation</u>

1. In a saucepan, heat oil, add chicken and cook until sealed and browned.

2. Add the water, apricots and sweet potato. Bring to a boil; simmer on lowered heat 15-20 minutes or until soft with minimal water left.

3. Puree the contents until smooth. It can be frozen for up to 6 weeks.

Peachy Chicken And Brown Rice

Ingredients

¼ cup of cooked brown rice

½ cup of cooked boneless chicken, chopped

1 ripe peach, pitted, peeled & baked or steamed

1 tablespoon of peach juice (apple or white grape juice)

I tablespoon of milk

2 tablespoon of wheat germ

Preparation

1. Combine all the ingredients.

2. Place in a food processor or blender and puree.

Chicken With Cheese& Pasta

Ingredients

½ cup of cottage cheese

½ cup cooked chicken, diced

1 cup of pasta, slightly cooled (pastina or ditalini)

¼ cup steamed broccoli

Dash pepper, basil and garlic powder

Preparation

1. Combine all ingredients and puree to desired consistency.

Turkey And Sweet Apples

<u>Ingredients</u>

1 medium sized apple, peeled, cored & diced

1 turkey breast fillet, uncooked & diced

1 cup sweet potato, peeled & diced

2 cups of water

<u>Preparation</u>

1. In a medium sized pot, combine all ingredients.

2. Bring to a gentle boil, lower heat and simmer 20 minutes or until the turkey pieces are cooked. Keep an eye on the level of water while simmering.

3. When meat is thoroughly cooked and apples are mushy, remove to a platter and let it cool.

4. Puree for your baby.

Chicken, Cheese And Broccoli

This delicious dish can be cooked in one pot.

<u>Ingredients</u>

1/4 cup of uncooked rice or couscous

1 cup shredded cooked chicken or 1 cooked chicken breast (boneless & skinless)

1/2 cup of chopped broccoli

2 cup of liquid (unsalted chicken or vegetable stock or water)

Cheddar or parmesan cheese, shredded

1 teaspoon of pesto (optional)

<u>Preparation</u>

1. Cut the chicken into cubes or pull the bone off if using a whole chicken.

2. Add together the chicken, broccoli, liquid and rice or couscous in a medium pot. Bring to a boil and then lower heat to simmer.

3. Cover and simmer 20 minutes or until the liquid is fully absorbed and the rice is thoroughly cooked.

4. If desired, add pesto and stir for extra flavor. Blend in a processor or serve warm with a sprinkle of cheese.

Chicken Corn With Cilantro

Cilantro becomes less potent when steamed; however, this is good for the baby's new palate. The cilantro's spiciness, the chicken's flavor and the corn's sweetness combine to make this dish irresistible for your kid.

Servings: 1 cup

<u>Ingredients</u>

1/2 cup cooked brown rice

2 tablespoons cilantro, stem and leaves

1 boneless, skinless chicken breast

1 cup water or chicken broth

2 tablespoons onions, sliced

1/4 cup corn, fresh or frozen

1 garlic clove

<u>Preparation</u>

1. Add all ingredients to a saucepan, except the corn and rice. Bring to a boil, simmer, cover and cook 5 minutes.

2. Add the corn and cook until chicken is cooked through, about 3 minutes.

3. Puree all ingredients, adding a tablespoon of broth at a time, until the right consistency for your baby is reached.

Fish Recipes (7months+)

Fish contains all that is necessary to develop a healthy nervous system: protein, B vitamins, calcium and selenium.

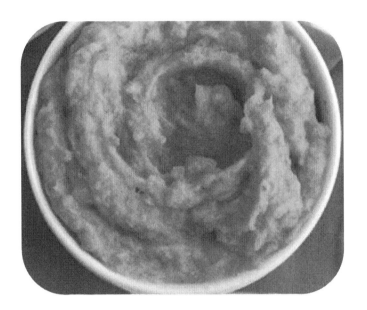

Salmon With Potatoes And Carrots

Salmon contains essential fatty acid that aid eye and brain development. This recipe has an abundant supply of protein, omega 3 fatty acids, iron, calcium, selenium and vitamins.

<u>Ingredients</u>

2 cups of chopped potato, peeled

4 ounces of salmon

½ cup shredded cheese

1 tablespoon of butter

1 cup carrot, peeled and sliced

31/2 tablespoons of milk

<u>Preparation</u>

1. Place the potatoes and carrots in a saucepan and cover with boiling water. Cook 20 minutes or until the veggies are soft.

2. Drain and mash with a baby food grinder or potato ricer to prevent lumps. Add 3 tablespoon of milk, cheese and butter while mashing.

3. Place the salmon in a dish, add ½ tablespoon of milk and microwave for 11/2 minutes.

4. Flake fish to ensure there are no bones and then mash with the potato and carrot mixture.

Fish And Spinach Meal
Give your baby the required vitamins and minerals with this fish recipe.

<u>Ingredients</u>

3-4 tablespoons of brown rice

Fresh white fish (Haddock or cod), debone & sliced

Spinach leaves, washed & chopped

<u>Preparation</u>

1. Wash the rice and drain. Add some water to a pan, bring to boil, add the rice and cook over low heat.

2. Let it simmer about 30 minutes. Stir constantly to prevent it from burning. In the last five minutes of cooking, add the fish and spinach.

3. Once the fish and veggies are cooked within a few minutes, remove from heat. Mix and ladle into baby's bowl

4. Let it to cool a little then feed your baby.

Salmon And Dill Dinner

From 10months up on account of the herb

Ingredients

4 oz. filet

1 tsp fresh dill, chopped

Chopped olives, optional

Preparation

1. Poach the salmon in simmering water for to 5 to10 minutes.

2. Puree with the fresh dill and olives and thin with water or plain yogurt.

Homemade Fish Stock

Ingredients

2/3 cups of dried anchovies, washed well to remove salt

1 liter of water

Fish bones or fish meat

Preparation

1. Drain the washed anchovies and set aside. Boil the water, add the fish and simmer over low heat.

2. Cover the pot and simmer again for about 30 minutes.

3. Strain the stock, cool and use. Freeze the remaining in ice cube trays.

Salmon & Broccoli Mash

This recipe is rich in calcium, omega 3 fatty acids, and beta-carotene.

Serves: 8 portions

<u>Ingredients</u>

31/2 ounces of fresh skinless salmon, filleted and de-boned (alternatively, use non-oily fish, such as haddock or cod)

1 small sweet potato, peeled & diced

3.4 fl oz milk

10 small broccoli florets

1/3 cup of water

<u>Preparation</u>

1. Boil the water in a saucepan and once boiling; add the broccoli and sweet potato, simmering 8-10 minutes until tender. Drain and mash.

2. Place the fish and milk in a pan and bring to a boil; simmer 8 minutes until cooked.

3. Mash the cooked fish with the milk, and then add mashed veggies.

4. Process to desired consistency for your baby. Add milk if necessary.

Steamed Pureed Fish With Green Veggies
<u>Ingredients</u>

1 potato, chopped

1 small zucchini, chopped

1 small fish fillet, debone and remove all skin

<u>Preparation</u>

1. Steam fish until cooked through, 5-10 minutes. Steam the potato until soft.

2. Add the cooked potato and fish to a blender and blend with formula or breast milk until smooth.

3. Steam the zucchini until tender; drain and blend until smooth. Add water, formula or breast milk to get your preferred consistency.

Cod Fillet With Vegetables

This fish dish will be good for your baby due to its fairly mild taste.

Ingredients

1 small carrot, grated

1 baby potato, peeled & chopped

1 cod fillet, skinned & sliced

1 small tomato, skinned &chopped

A dash of pepper

Butter

Bay leaf

Preparation

1. Place the veggies in a pan of water, cover and bring to a boil. Lower heat and simmer 15 minutes or until tender

2. Place the fillet in another pan and add pepper, bay leaf and pour some milk over it. Poach fish until it flakes easily, about 5 minutes. Discard the bay leaf.

3. Melt the butter in a pan and sauté the tomato until mushy. Add in the flaked fish and stir.

4. Add in the cooked veggies and mash with a mouli until the right consistency is obtained. Add some liquid, if necessary.

Cod, Broccoli & Sweet Potato Mix

Broccoli is a good source of calcium so give your baby often.

<u>Ingredients</u>

1 small sweet potato, skinned& cut into bite-sizes

I small cod fillet, deboned & skinned

Few florets of broccoli, washed well

<u>Preparation</u>

1. Place the cut potato and broccoli florets in the steamer and steam 20 to 25 minutes.

2. Add the cod and steam again for another 10 minutes. Mash to the right consistency.

Sardine And Avocado Spread

A rich, healthy and filling snack from 10 months up

<u>Ingredients</u>

½ of an avocado

2 canned sardines in oil, drained& mashed well

1 teaspoon of lemon juice

<u>Preparation</u>

1. Mash the ingredients together.

2. Use as a dip or toast topper.

Fish, Sweet Potato And Broccoli Mash

Babies can take fish when mixed with vegetables, especially sole, on account of its tenderness.

Servings: 3 portions

Ingredients

2 broccoli florets, cut into small pieces

½ cup (about 7oz) sweet potato, peeled & diced

4 ounce sole fillet, skinned & cut into strips

½ cup of milk

2 tablespoon shredded cheese

Preparation

1. Steam the sweet potato and broccoli covered until tender, for 6 to 8 minutes.

2. Meanwhile, place the fish in a pan, pour the milk over it and cook for 2 minutes until it flakes easily.

3. Remove from heat and add the cheese, stirring until melted. Add the fish mixture and vegetables and puree in a blender.

4. Freeze in individual portions or cover and refrigerate. Serve puree by heating and stirring in a saucepan or microwave until hot. Add more milk if necessary. Let it cool a bit and then serve baby.

Red Peppered Plaice In Orange Juice

Ingredients

1 small fillet plaice

1 baby potato skinned & cubed

½ red pepper, finely chopped

Grated cheddar cheese

½ a carrot peeled & diced

Fresh orange juice

Chopped parsley as seasoning

Butter

Preparation

1. Steam the vegetables until tender.

2. Meanwhile, place the fish in a gratin dish and then pour the orange juice over it. Top with cheese and butter.

3. Cover with foil paper, place in a preheated oven and bake 20 minutes.

4. Remove fish from oven, flake and remove any bones. Add the veggies and its juices to a blender and blend to a coarse or smooth puree, depending on preference.

Stir- Fried Cod With Vegetables

<u>Ingredients</u>

A handful of rice grains

1 small piece of boneless cod, diced

½ of a small white onion, finely chopped

1 tablespoon of butter

A handful of cabbage

½ cup of vegetable stock

1 small carrot, cubed

<u>Preparation</u>

1. Stir-fry the onion in oil. Add the fillet and cook about 4 minutes.

2. add all the other ingredients and simmer for 20 minutes or until rice and vegetables are soft.

3. Puree to desired consistency. If necessary, add more stock.

Tofu Recipes (9 Months+)

Tofu is a byproduct of Soya beans and contains protein, iron and calcium. However, the complexity of its protein may upset a baby's immature stomach. Therefore, your baby must be at least 9 months old before you introduce tofu to him or her. In addition, soy is a potential allergen food so do not offer your baby if he has soy allergy.

Unused tofu can be stored in an airtight container for up to 7 days, but the water must be changed daily. Tofu should retain the freshness, it mustn't smell sour.

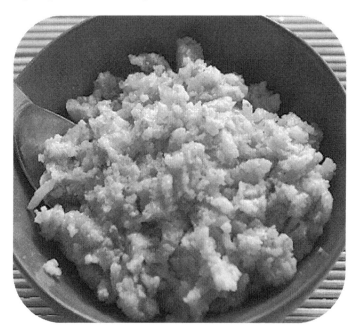

Creamed Pumpkin With Tofu

Tofu combines well with fruits and vegetables.

<u>Ingredients</u>

1 small pumpkin, peeled &diced

¼ cup of tofu

3 ounce full fat milk

1 tablespoon fresh orange juice

<u>Preparation</u>

1. Steam parsnips for about 10 minutes or until soft. In another bowl, drain the tofu piece and crumble.

2. For a younger baby, blend the parsnip pieces, the tofu and juice together until smooth. Add milk, a little at a time, to make a smooth but thick puree.

3. Serve your baby. If too thick, add more milk. (Pumpkin may be substituted with parsnip or melon slice)

Tofu Nuggets
<u>Ingredients</u>

1 teaspoon of paprika

1 package of firm tofu, cut in cubes

¼ cup of flour

2 egg yolks

1 teaspoon of garlic powder

1 cup bread crumb or fine cracker

Dash pepper

<u>Preparation</u>

1. Set the oven to 350 degrees F. Beat the eggs onto a dish and put the flour in a plate. Put the remaining ingredients in another dish.

2. Coat each piece of the tofu in flour, then the egg yolk and finally the rest of the ingredients.

3. Bake for 15 to 20 minutes at 350 degrees F until the tofu is crisp.

4. Serve with ketchup or with pureed fruit.

Scrambled Tofu With Leek And Peas
<u>Ingredients</u>

½ tofu piece crumbled

2 tablespoon of green peas

1 teaspoon red onion, finely diced

1 tbsp tomato, diced

White of leek, chopped

Cumin or basil leaf, for seasoning

Olive oil

<u>Preparation</u>

1. In a pan, sauté onion in olive oil for 3 minutes. Add the basil leaf or cumin seeds.

2. Now add leek and peas and cook another 5 minutes. Add the tomato and keep cooking until the vegetables are soft.

3. Add crumbled tofu and cook for 5 minutes, stirring occasionally.

4. Puree to a thick paste for younger babies but leave it coarse for older ones. Serve while warm.

Silken Tofu With Fresh Chives

Ingredients

1 avocado, diced

½ cup silken tofu

½ cup fresh chives, chopped

Preparation

1. Mash the tofu; add in the chives and mix well.

2. Refrigerate and serve.

Tofu With Brown Rice

Tofu has a natural aroma; and when combined with brown rice, the flavor becomes more distinct. You can make this recipe soupier by adding more water or enjoy in its pudding-like texture.

Ingredients

½ block of silken tofu

2-3 tablespoons of brown rice grounded

Filtered water

Preparation

1. Steam tofu 5 to 7 minutes and set aside with the water.

2. Cook the rice in water until done or for about 20 minutes.

3. Add the tofu pieces to the rice and serve your baby.

Lentils, Tomatoes & Vegetables (9-12 Months)

Lentils are high in protein and fiber. They are considered as gassy foods but most parents love them because they are generally non allergy-causing. Presoaking overnight minimizes gassiness and saves up on cooking time.

Use fresh tomatoes when making homemade baby food. Their skin must be intact with no signs of bruising. Tomatoes are very acidic; therefore, they are recommended for babies that are least 9 months old.

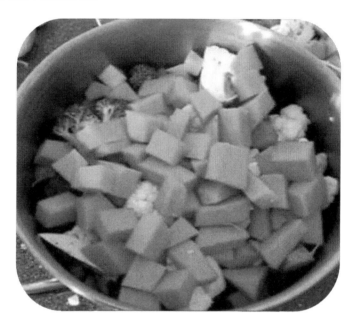

Pureed Lentils
<u>Ingredients</u>

2 tablespoons red lentils

½ carrot, diced

I tablespoon onion, chopped

½ teaspoon garlic

½ teaspoon ginger

1 teaspoon of oil

Water for cooking

Parsley or coriander, chopped

Cumin powder and/or pepper (optional)

<u>Preparation</u>

1. Sauté onion, carrots, ginger, and garlic in the oil for 10 minutes until the carrots are tender.

2. Add the water and lentils and cook another 20 minutes or until soft.

3. Season with herbs and spices. Blend everything to a puree form. To thin, add boiled water or milk and serve your baby.

4. (Serve an older baby with cooked pasta or rice).

Adzuki Brown Rice

Adzuki beans are good for the kidneys. These small reddish-brown beans should be soaked for 5 hours or better still, overnight, with the water thrown away before cooking. This recipe's quantity is small so 1 hour of pre-soaking will do.

<u>Ingredients</u>

2-3 tablespoons of brown rice

2 tablespoons adzuki beans

Small ginger piece

1 cup water

<u>Preparation</u>

1. Combine the beans, ginger and water in a pot and bring to a boil. Cook for 15-20 minutes, checking the water as it cooks and adding more water if needed.

2. Add the rice to the cooked beans and cook until soft. Remove the ginger piece, mash or blend and serve.

Lentils With Carrots And Tomatoes

These foods are antioxidants. For great fiber, iron and folate, use quick cooking lentils.

<u>Ingredients</u>

2/3 cup of red lentils

1 cup canned coconut milk

2 skinned tomatoes, deseeded & chopped

2 carrots, grated

1tbsp olive oil

¼ teaspoon ground coriander

¼ teaspoon ground cumin

1 ¼ vegetable stock

<u>Preparation</u>

1. Sauté the carrots and tomatoes in oil for about 5 minutes until soft. Add the spices, stir and cook 30 seconds.

2. Add lentils, coconut milk and stock. Boil and simmer 20 minutes until the lentils are soft.

3. Puree everything or mash for more texture.

Veggie Lasagna Puree
For babies without diary/wheat allergies

Your baby will love the lasagna flavor in this puree recipe. From tomato paste, mix of healthy veggies and spices to enrich the taste, your baby will ask for more!

<u>Ingredients</u>

1 cup zucchini (and/or peas, eggplant, spinach, etc.), chopped

2 tablespoons organic tomato paste

2 carrots, chopped

½ onion, diced

1 tablespoon extra-virgin olive oil

2 tablespoons ricotta cheese

1 cup vegetable or chicken stock

Pinch garlic powder or 1 small garlic clove

Pinch of dried oregano

½ cup pasta (of choice)

1 teaspoon Parmesan cheese, grated

<u>Preparation</u>

1. Cook all the ingredients until soft and then puree until smooth.

Simple Tomato Sauce
<u>Ingredient</u>

5 large tomatoes, washed & diced

1/2 medium sized onion, diced

1 clove of garlic, finely minced

1 tablespoon olive oil

2 tablespoons of fresh basil, chopped

Bay, rosemary, oregano or any other herbs

3 cups of water

<u>Preparation</u>

1. In a medium saucepan, heat the olive oil. Add onion and garlic and cook until onion is translucent

2. Now add water and tomatoes, stir and bring mixture to a boil

3. Lower heat and partially cover pot. Simmer 40 minutes, stirring occasionally.

4. Add herbs of choice and simmer for 5 more minutes. Puree sauce until smooth.

5. Serve over pasta with baby meatballs and parmesan cheese, grated.

Serving Ideas

1. Make "pizza" for your baby by spreading some sauce on a slice of bread and top it with shredded mozzarella. You can also top with some diced olives, ham, pineapple and spinach. Place in an oven or toaster oven until the bread is crispy and cheese melts.

2. Pour some warm sauce over grilled diced zucchini, squash and/or eggplant.

Tomatoey Rice

Ingredients

1½ cups uncooked rice (not instant)

1 cup tomato sauce

2 1/2 cups vegetable or chicken broth

1/4 onion, finely diced

2 tablespoons vegetable oil

4 teaspoon of garlic powder or 2 cloves garlic, grated or minced

Preparation

1. Heat oil in a pan over medium heat. Add onion and cook until soft and translucent, about 1 minute.

2. Add the rice and cook about 5 minutes until rice is golden brown.

3. Add garlic, stirring to coat with oil then add the tomato sauce and broth.

4. Bring to a boil, lower heat, cover and simmer 20 minutes on low heat.

5. Open lid and fluff with a fork

Yellow Pea Soup

A delicious soup that is packed with the goodness of protein

Ingredients

2 tablespoons dried yellow split lentil

1 teaspoon of chopped onion

½ cup carrot, peeled& chopped

Celery, peeled & chopped

½ sweet potato, peeled & cubed

2 tablespoons cream corn

Dash of pepper

Preparation

1. Boil the lentil until tender. Add the veggies and simmer until vegetables are soft, about an hour and half.

2. Drain some of the water if necessary and then puree until creamy and smooth.

3. For added flavor, sauté the onion with the thyme and bay leaf in a little olive oil.

Broccoli With Tomatoes And Almonds

This vegetarian meal is a good source of beta-carotene, vitamin E, calcium, and vitamin C.

Ingredients

2 tablespoons of chopped tomatoes

2 broccoli florets

¼ cup flaked almonds, toasted lightly & finely ground

1. Place the florets in a steamer and steam until tender.

2. Add to a blender and the tomatoes as well and blend well.

3. Add the ground almonds, stir and serve.

Spinach And Lentils

Ingredients

15g fresh spinach chopped

1 tablespoon of white rice

1/8 cup of red or yellow lentils, soaked for 30 minutes

Vegetable oil

Homemade vegetable stock or water

Pinch coriander powder

Pinch turmeric powder

½ of a small tomato, skinned & chopped (optional)

Preparation

1. Combine the rice, lentils, oil, spices and stock or water in a pan and bring to a boil.

2. Let it simmer for 11/2 hours or until the rice and lentils are soft, stirring often.

3. Add in the spinach and tomato, stir and cook 2 minutes. Puree the mixture until smooth and thick. (As your baby grows older, adjust the texture accordingly)

4. Cool a little and then serve.

Parsnip, Carrot And Chickpea Mix
<u>Ingredients</u>

1 carrot, peeled& chopped coarsely

2 cups water, crushed ginger

½ parsnip, peeled &chopped

½ can or pre-boiled chickpeas (drained &rinsed)

Grated parsley cheese, optional,

<u>Preparation</u>

1. Combine vegetables and water in a pot and bring to the boil. Simmer 8 minutes over low heat.

2. Add the ginger, chickpeas, and cook 10 more minutes or until the veggies are tender. Remove and cool slightly.

3. Take out the ginger piece; puree the veggies and chickpeas, adding the cooking liquid until smooth.

4. Garnish with cheese and parsley

Lentil And Veggie Puree
This recipe is not only simple and nutritious, but yummy and satisfying as well.

<u>Ingredients</u>

Red or yellow lentils

Small ginger piece, white part of the leek chopped off

Carrot

Sweet potato

Pinch of turmeric powder

Bay leaf for flavor

Butter

Preparation

1. Melt the butter in a pan and then add the, ginger, leeks and bay leaf. Sauté for 3-4 minutes and then add the chopped carrots, lentils and turmeric powder, stirring and cooking for another 5 minutes.

2. Add the sweet potatoes and water then simmer over low heat until lentils and veggies are tender.

3. Remove the bay leaf and piece of ginger, mash or blend the mixture to a puree. (Serve older babies as it is).

Homemade Vegetable Stock
Ingredients

1 large carrot, peeled &diced

1 stick celery, peeled & chopped

White onion

Olive oil

Garlic clove

Bay leaf

1 ginger slice

1 liter water

Preparation

1. Sauté the garlic and onion in the oil. Add all other ingredients and cover with water.

2. Let it boil then cover and simmer1 hour.

3. Remove the bay leaf and ginger and puree or blend the stock. Serve and freeze what is left in ice cube trays.

Leek, Cauliflower& Sweet Potato Puree
Servings: 12-24 portions

Ingredients

¼ large leek, white part, sliced finely

1tablespoon of butter

1 cup of cauliflower, broken into floret

2 cups sweet potato

1/3 cup grated cheese

1 cup boiling water

Preparation

1. Heat the butter in a pan and sauté the leek until soft.

2. Add the sweet potato and boiling water and cook 5 minutes.

3. Add the cauliflower, cover and cook another 5 minutes.

4. Add the cheese and puree the mixture.

Egg Recipes (9 Months +)

Eggs are packed with protein and vitamins. However, they are generally allergens, particularly the whites. It is advisable to offer whole egg to your baby only when he or she turns a year old.

Egg yolk is safe at 9 months though. Cook eggs for babies by preparing scrambled eggs on low heat. Do not give them hard boiled eggs as they will be unable to properly digest them at 9 months. Wait until they are at least a year. Cook eggs until the white and yolk are solid.

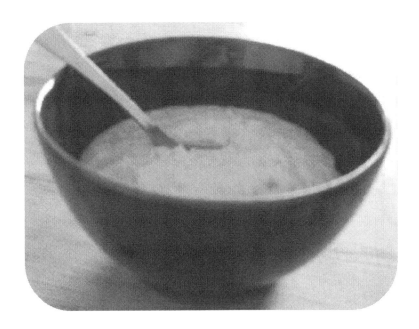

Parsley & Broccoli Omelet
<u>Ingredients</u>

2 egg (whites separated)

4 tablespoon full fat milk

Unsalted butter

Egg yolk

Parsley, finely chopped

Broccoli, finely cut

Preparation

1. Warm the butter in a skillet and fry the broccoli for about 1 or 2 minutes.

2. In a mixing bowl, break the egg without the white, whisk in the milk and add the parsley, beating well. Add this mixture to the skillet and cook on one side.

3. Flip and cook for 1 more minute and then remove with a spatula and serve.

Egg With Chive
From 12 months

Ingredients

Hard boil egg

¼ teaspoon of chives, finely chopped

Plain yogurt

Paprika, optional

Preparation

1. Puree egg or yolk with chives and paprika, if using.

2. Thin with plain yogurt.

Egg And Quinoa
Ingredients

¼ cup of quinoa

1 tablespoon of diced onion

1 small piece of pumpkin diced

Egg yolk scrambled in a little butter

1½ cups of water

Preparation

1. Bring water to boil, add the quinoa and onion and simmer on lower heat for 15 minutes.

2. Add pumpkin and keep cooking on low heat for 10 more minutes until the vegetable is soft. Add the scrambled egg and stir thoroughly.

3. Puree until smooth or coarse, according to your baby's taste.

Scrambled Eggs And Ham
From 12 months

Ingredients

3-4 large eggs

Boiled ham, diced

Shredded cheddar cheese

Preparation

1. In a small bowl, beat in the eggs and add the diced cooked ham.

2. Preheat a pan over medium heat. Cook the egg mixture in a preheated pan, stirring often until cooked through.

3. Sprinkle with cheddar cheese and serve.

Egg Yolk Puree

Introduce egg yolk with baby's favorite fruit or vegetable puree such as peach, avocado, pear, sweet potato or banana purees.

Ingredients

1 or 2 egg yolks

Any fruit or vegetable puree

1 to 2 tablespoon of milk (optional)

Preparation

1. Boil the egg. Remove the shell and scoop the hardened yolk out of the boiled egg.

2. Mash and add the fruit puree of choice.

Scrambled Eggs Cauliflower Puree
From 12 months

Scrambled eggs are so soft they can never be considered as a choking hazard. Even older babies can pick them up with a big grasp.

Servings: 3-4

Ingredients

3-4 large eggs

1 cup head of cauliflower, boiled or steamed or boiled

3-4 tablespoons of liquid (steam pot water, formula or breast milk)

Preparation

1. Puree the cauliflower with the liquid.

2. In a small bowl, beat in the eggs and add the pureed cauliflower. Preheat a pan over medium heat

3. Cook the egg mixture in a preheated pan, stirring often until cooked through.

4. Freeze the leftovers.

Cheese Eggs & Spinach
From 12 months

Servings: 3-4

Ingredients

3-4 large eggs

1 handful of fresh spinach, chopped into medium-size pieces

A sprinkle of cheddar or mozzarella cheese (grated)

Preparation

1. Add chopped spinach to a preheated a pan and cook until soft.

2. In a small bowl, beat in eggs and add to pan.

3. Cook and stir constantly, until cooked through

4. Sprinkle with cheese and serve

Eggs & Eggplant Combo

From 12 months

Ingredients

3-4 large eggs

About 1 cup eggplant, peeled and diced

Preparation

1. In a covered pan, sauté the eggplant with a little vegetable oil over medium heat until very soft.

2. Puree the sautéed eggplant or leave as is.

3. In a small bowl, beat in the eggs and add the pureed eggplant or the very soft one.

4. Preheat a pan over medium heat. Cook the egg mixture in a preheated pan, stirring often until cooked through.

Desserts (6-7months+)

Serves: 1 portion

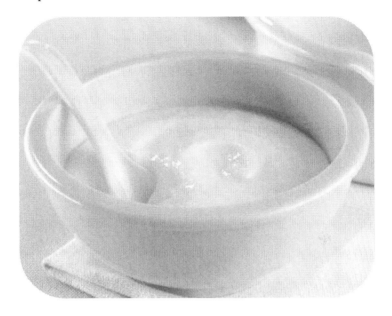

Lemony Rice Pudding

Your traditional rice pudding with a lemony twist is a good source of vitamins B and calcium.

<u>Ingredients</u>

1/8 cup of pudding rice

2-3 small strips of lemon peel

11/4 cup full cream milk

Pinch ground cinnamon, optional

<u>Preparation</u>

1. Combine the milk, rice and lemon peel in a pan and heat gently for 25 minutes or until the rice is soft, stirring constantly.

2. Take out the lemon peel and stir. Add the ground cinnamon if using.

Coco Egg Custard

The inclusion of coconut's creamy favor livens up this traditional egg custard recipe for your baby.

Ingredients

1 egg

1-2 drops of vanilla essence

3.4 fl.oz reduced-fat canned coconut milk

1 tablespoon of apricot puree

Preparation

1. Add together all ingredients and mix well.

2. Pour into two ramekins or teacups and steam for 10 minutes until set.

3. it's important that this dish is thoroughly heated until piping hot, so that the eggs are well cooked. Chill before serving.

Chocolaty Banana Custard

Mashed banana and chocolate is deliciously combined to make this sweet custard. This dish is packed with calcium and B vitamins.

Ingredients

1 small banana

1 teaspoon of corn-flour

1 teaspoon drinking chocolate (granules or powder)

3.4 oz fl milk or formula

1. Combine the corn-flour, milk and chocolate powder in a bowl. Place in a microwave and heat for 1-2 minutes until thickened.

2. Alternatively, gently heat on the hob and stir constantly. Mash the banana and serve it with the custard.

Brown Rice Pudding

Ingredients

1 tablespoon of brown rice

4-5 oz formula or breast milk

1 small apple pureed

Pinch of cinnamon, ground

Handful of figs, apricots or raisins

Butter

Filtered water, if necessary

Pinch nutmeg

Brown sugar, for taste

Preparation

1. Ground the brown rice until it is in powdery form. Add some milk and mix well. Add the remaining milk and cook until creamy, about 10 minutes.

2. Add the pureed apple, figs, butter, sugar, nutmeg and cinnamon powder and cook for another 30minutes.

3. Simmer over low flame until the milk is absorbed and mixture forms pudding- like texture. Serve warm or cold.

Pear Dessert

This fruity treat contains vitamin C and is a good source of calcium and B vitamins.

Ingredients

1 tablespoon of apple juice

1 ripe pear, peeled& sliced

1 tablespoon of 8% fat fromage frais

Pinch of cinnamon

Preparation

1. Simmer the pear in the apple juice gently until soft, about 5 minutes.

2. Let it cool, sieve and then add the fromage frais and cinnamon.

Creamy Apricot Dessert

This simple dessert takes seconds to prepare and is a good source of calcium and beta-carotene.

Ingredients

4 tablespoons of Greek yoghurt

½ cup of mascarpone cheese

3 tablespoon of apricot puree (prepared from canned & drained apricots in unsweetened fruit juice)

Preparation

1. Whisk the cheese and yoghurt together, add the apricot puree and whisk again.

2. Eat with a spoon or Use as dip for cut grapes.

Apple Cinnamon Yoghurt
Serves: 2 portions

Ingredients

3 tablespoons of natural Greek yoghurt

2 tablespoons of puree apple

Pinch of cinnamon

Preparation

1. Add together the apple puree and cinnamon yoghurt until desired sweetness is attained.

Apricot Apple Dessert
A simple and fruity dessert containing vitamin C and beta-carotene

Ingredients

1/3 cup soft dried apricots, chopped roughly

1 apple, peeled & chopped roughly

3.4 oz fl water

Preparation

1. Place the apricots in a saucepan, add the water and simmer 5 minutes.

2. Add the apple and cook on low until soft.

3. Puree to desired consistency for your baby.

Banana, Grape And Yogurt Dessert

This fruity pudding will provide your baby with vitamin C and calcium

<u>Ingredients</u>

½ cup cottage cheese

¼ cup of grapes

½ cup 8% fat fromage frais

½ of a banana

<u>Preparation</u>

1. Place all ingredients in a food processor or blender and puree until smooth.

Teething And Pick Up Foods

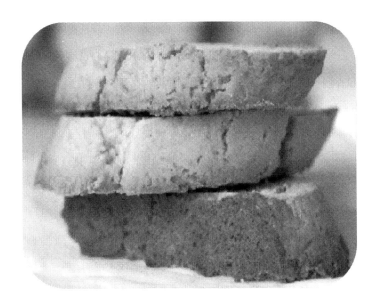

DIY Teething Rusks

Make teething rusks for your baby to chew on. They are so easy and bring great delight to babies when cutting new teeth.

<u>Ingredients</u>

5 slices of whole-meal stale bread

<u>Preparation</u>

1. Remove the crusts and cut bread into fingers.

2. Place the bread on a baking sheet and bake slowly until the bread fingers are hard and dry or for 1 hour at 125°C.

3. Cool and store in a tight-fitting container.

Apple And Mango Ice Delights

These delicious ice blocks will make for an enjoyable mid-afternoon snack and soothe sore gums as well.

Ingredients

1 medium apple, peeled, cored &diced

1 medium mango, peeled

Preparation

1. Cut off the mango flesh and mash with in a small bowl until thoroughly smooth.

2. Half fill all the blocks in an1 x ice cube tray with the mango puree. Freeze until frozen solid, about 2 hours.

3. In a saucepan, place the apples and just cover with water. Over a medium-high heat, bring to a boil and simmer on medium until cooked through, about 5 minutes.

3. In a blender, puree apples with 1/4 cup of the cooking water. Remove the frozen mango from the ice cube tray, and fill all the blocks with the apple puree. Freeze again until solid, about 2 hours.

4. Remove blocks from tray; place one of it in a fruit net. Using the back of a spoon, bang gently to soften a little and offer your baby.

Mashed Banana Teething Biscuits
Ingredients

1¾ cups of whole-meal flour

1 cup of mashed bananas

2 eggs

1/4 cup brown sugar

2 teaspoons of baking powder

1/2 cup vegetable oil

1/2 teaspoons baking soda

<u>Preparation</u>

1. Preheat the oven to 180°C. Place baking paper on a slice tray and set aside.

2. Combine all ingredients in a bowl until well mixed. Pour into slice tin and bake 1 hour.

3. Remove, let it cool and then slice into sticks. Lay on baking paper.

4. Reduce the oven temperature to 150°C and bake another1 hour.

Breakfast Treat
This pick up food is good for the baby. Baby picks up the food, chews and swallows it

7-8 months

<u>Ingredients</u>

½ of a small banana

2 tablespoon of plain yoghurt

2 tablespoon of ripe peach, peeled& cut into bite-sized pieces

2 tablespoon baby oatmeal or ground oatmeal

<u>Preparation</u>

1. Mash together the yoghurt and banana and then add the peach pieces. Stir until well coated.

2. Roll in the ground oatmeal until well coated and easy to pick up.

Miscellaneous Baby Meals (7months up)

Trying new flavors and textures is one way to wean your baby successfully. These simple, nutritious recipes will make it easier for you to do.

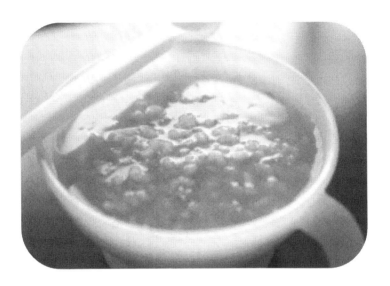

Sweet Potato Cheese Mash

Packed with beta-carotene, this colorful mash also contains vitamin C and calcium.

<u>Ingredients</u>

1 medium carrot, peeled & diced

4 oz sweet potato, peeled & diced

¼ cup of cheddar cheese, grated

<u>Preparation</u>

1. Boil the vegetables in a pan until just tender.

2. Add to a food processor and puree along with the cheese.

Avocado And Yoghurt Dip

Mashed avocado, a great source of monounsaturated fat, also works well as a dip.

Ingredients

½ of a ripe avocado

1 tbsp yoghurt

1 tsp lemon juice

Preparation

1. Blend all the ingredients together in a blender.

Cottage Cheese Pea Mash

Light, easy to prepare, simple and full of goodness.

Ingredients

1/3 cup of frozen peas

½ cup low salt cottage cheese

Preparation

1. Cook the peas until just tender. Remove from heat.

2. Puree along with to the cottage cheese. Serve with bread fingers or rice cakes.

Lentil Dahl With Orange

This colorful, wholesome mixture has vitamin C iron and beta-carotene.

Ingredients

½ cup of lentils

11/4 cups of water

3tablespoons of orange juice

Pinch of cinnamon

Preparation

1. Place the lentils in a pan and pour water over it, cover and cook gently until the lentils are soft, about 20 minutes.

2. Drain slightly with a sieve and return the drained lentils to pan.

3. Add the orange juice and cinnamon, stir and return to the heat for a few seconds.

Eggs With Whole-Meal Bread

This is a good stand-by meal that is loved by most babies.

Ingredients

1 egg, well beaten

1 slice of soft whole-meal bread

A little butter or oil

Preparation

1. Heat the butter in a pan. Dip the bread in the well-beaten egg, turning to coat well.

2. Place in the hot fat carefully and fry on both sides until golden brown.

3. Remove from heat, place fried bread on kitchen paper to absorb surplus oil and then cut into tiny fingers.

4. Serve along with slices of Satsuma or tomato, or sprinkled with some cinnamon.

Mediterranean Ratatouille

A lovely medley of veggies your baby will love.

Ingredients

1 small zucchini, diced

1 small yellow or red pepper, seeded &diced

4 tomatoes, skinned & seeded

1 teaspoon of olive oil

Few slices of eggplant, diced

½ of a small onion, chopped finely

Preparation

1. Fry the onion lightly in the oil. Add all the other veggies and stir.

2. Cover, lower heat and cook about 30 minutes or until the veggies are tender.

3. Puree or mash to desired consistency for your baby.

Lamb With Apple

This yummy mix of fruit and meat contains vitamins B and C and is also an excellent source of iron.

Ingredients

7 ounce of lamb, minced

7 tablespoons unsweetened apple juice

1 cooking apple, grated

½ tsp of dried tarragon

1 small zucchini, diced

Pinch ground cinnamon

Preparation

1. In a pan, cook the lamb in its own fat until thoroughly browned. Drain off the fat.

2. Return the minced lamb to the pan and add the apple, zucchini and apple juice. Stir well, cover and cook 15 minutes.

3. Add the tarragon and cinnamon, stir and simmer another 5 minutes. Blend lightly to remove large lumps. Serve with mashed potato.

Quinoa Ratatouille
9-12 Months

This baby food quinoa ratatouille is stuffed with, eggplant, zucchini, tomato, squash, sweet peppers, and of course, quinoa. Full of protein, antioxidants, fiber and iron, it is a quick cook with tiny seeds for your baby will eat easily.

Ingredients

¼ cup of quinoa

1 cup zucchini, diced

1 tomato, chopped

1 tablespoon olive oil

1 pinch thyme leaves, dried

¼ medium onion, diced

½ cup red bell or green pepper, diced

2 tablespoons tomato paste

1 cup eggplant, diced

1 cup of vegetable broth

1-2 tablespoons of grated Parmesan cheese (optional)

1 pinch garlic (fresh or powdered)

Fresh basil and/or parsley (optional)

Preparation

1. Heat the olive oil in a saucepan over medium heat. Add the onion and cook about 5 minutes or until soft.

2. Add the garlic, eggplant, thyme, zucchini, sweet pepper, tomato paste, quinoa, tomato and vegetable broth, stir and bring to a simmer.

3. Lower heat, cover and cook for 15-20 minutes or until the quinoa 'shoots out" and the veggies are tender. If necessary, add more broth during cooking.

4. Remove from heat and add the fresh herbs and cheese, stirring well.

5. Puree in a food processor or blender until the desired consistency is achieved, add extra water or vegetable broth if needed.

Banana, Yoghurt And Honey Porridge
From 12 months

A dash of sweet honey, a little banana and yoghurt is all it takes to add zest to this recipe. It is packed with the necessary nutrients such as calcium for great bones and teeth, and vitamins A, B6, C, magnesium, zinc and iron.

Ingredients

1/4 cup rolled oats

1/4 cup plain yoghurt

1/3 banana, mashed

1/3 cup milk, formula, water or breast milk

1 teaspoon honey

Preparation

1. In a saucepan, place all the ingredients and bring to a boil.

2. Simmer 5minutes until soft, stirring often. Let it cool and serve warm.

Preparation

1. Add oil in a saucepan, add onion and cook over medium heat until soft.

2. Stir in oregano and garlic, add veggies, carrots, stock and tomato paste. Stir well and bring to a boil.

3. Add the pasta. Cover and cook until carrots are tender, 10-15 minutes.

4. Remove from heat once all the vegetables are tender; add the Parmesan and ricotta cheese, stirring well.

5. Let it cool and puree until smooth. Gradually add the cooking liquid until you get the right consistency.

Spicy Curried Chicken With Fruits
12-18 Months

Tempt your baby's palate with this spicy chicken meal

<u>Ingredients</u>

2 tablespoons of sunflower oil

1 chicken breast, cubed

1 tablespoon of tomato paste

1 small shallot, chopped finely

2, dried apricot, chopped

7 ounces butternut squash, chopped & peeled

2 teaspoon of mild korma curry taste

2/3 cup of unsalted chicken stock

<u>Preparation</u>

1. Sauté the shallot in oil for about 4 minutes.

2. Add the chicken and sauté until white on the outside.

3. Add the curry taste and stir well. Add the remaining ingredients and simmer 10 minutes.

4. Add everything to a blender or food processor and puree.

Squashy Wheels
8-10 Months

Your baby will love this yummy snack. It is quick and easy.

<u>Ingredients</u>

4-5 small yellow squash, thinly sliced (1/4 inch)

3/4 cup bread crumbs (panko bread crumbs)

3 tablespoons of olive oil

3/4 cup Parmesan cheese, grated

1/2 teaspoon pepper

Parsley

<u>Preparation</u>

1. Preheat oven to 450° F. Combine breadcrumbs, parmesan cheese and pepper in a shallow bowl.

2. In a separate bowl, place the squash and toss lightly with olive oil.

3. Dredge the sliced squash in the bread crumb mixture to coat on all sides.

4. Remove to a parchment lined baking sheet and bake until golden, 25-30 minutes.

5. Remove from oven and sprinkle with parsley.

17936007R00063

Printed in Great Britain
by Amazon